WORKOUT MOTIVATION

The Ultimate Guide on How to Develop a Fitness Mindset, Learn the Effective Strategies and Tips on How to Stay Motivated For Fitness

Descrierea CIP a Bibliotecii Naţionale a României
CLIFF GUNTER
   WORKOUT MOTIVATION. The Ultimate Guide on How to Develop a Fitness Mindset, Learn the Effective Strategies and Tips on How to Stay Motivated For Fitness / Cliff Gunter – Bucharest: Editura My Ebook, 2021
   ISBN

CLIFF GUNTER

WORKOUT MOTIVATION
The Ultimate Guide on How to Develop a Fitness Mindset, Learn the Effective Strategies and Tips on How to Stay Motivated For Fitness

My Ebook Publishing House
Bucharest, 2021

TABLE OF CONTENTS

Foreword 7

Chapter 1: *Basics On Fitness* 9

Chapter 2: *The Condition Of Peoples Health These Days* 13

Chapter 3: *What Is True Fitness* 18

Chapter 4: *What Is The Empowered Fitness Mindset....* 22

Chapter 5: *Traditional Fitness Ideas vs. New Age Ideas* 26

Chapter 6: *What Does Empowerment for Fitness Mean to You* 29

Chapter 7: *Why Adopt The Empowerment Mindset For Fitness* 33

Chapter 8: *Tips For Becoming Empowered For Fitness* 36

Chapter 9: *The Good And Bad About The Empowerment Mindset For Fitness* 39

Chapter 10: *Conclusion* 43

FOREWORD

When it comes to fitness, you don't need to be a runner or aspire to be an athlete to start improving your overall fitness condition. If you want to be physically fit, you need full determination and focus on what you want to achieve in order for you to be successful. Get all the info you need here.

CHAPTER 1

BASICS ON FITNESS

Synopsis

With the alarming rates of diseases that affect people nowadays, it is important for people to consider improving their physical fitness.

Unfortunately, with the wide variety of foods that surround the market at present, it can be challenging for some to avoid or neglect their cravings on their favorite foods.

However, what they don't know is that not all foods are healthy for improving one's fitness. Some of them can cause health risks, which are not a good thing most particularly if you aim to be physically fit. That is why it is wise for everyone to choose healthy foods wisely.

The Basics

If you have decided to take up exercising to improve your fitness, well, congratulations! It is because empowering your fitness is the most vital step that will lead you to the "new" you! Now, the only thing that you should do is to stick with your plan and learn the basics of fitness.

There are various reasons why some people decide to incorporate physical fitness in their lives. Whether you are aiming to lose your weight, gain size or enhance you well-being, empowering your fitness can be the key for a healthier living.

The basics of fitness revolve around improving your nutrition and doing exercises. In order for you to achieve success in improving your fitness, you need to exert 100% effort and commitment. When you think of fitness, it is vital for you to take a peek at the big picture.

You have to take note that fitness is not just about endurance, strength or fat content, but also it's the combination of those factors. You can be strong, but you have no endurance. You may have endurance, but you might be less flexible.

In fitness, you need to aim for balance. There are five components that make a good fitness. Proficiency in these components will give you long- term benefits and value to your overall well-being and fitness. These components are as follows:

- *Aerobic Endurance* - repetitive or rhythmic activities placed an increase oxygen demand on your body systems, lungs, and heart. Big muscle groups can be used in various activities including cycling, jogging or walking. The aim of this component is to train other muscles and heart to use oxygen efficiently, which permits exercise to continue for a long period of time.

- *Muscular Strength* - It is the capacity of the muscles of your body to produce a huge amount of force to utilize anaerobic energy. This energy produces a short term burst of energy and will not require oxygen. Anaerobic energy comes after the carbohydrates were burned, which is needed in replenishing the system.

- *Muscular Endurance* - It is the measure of how your muscles can repetitively generate force to maintain the activity. This is use of the raw strengths. When compared other components, this combines both anaerobic and aerobic energy.

- *Flexibility* - This is ability of a person to stretch. You can increase your flexibility through stretching elastic fibers beyond their limits and maintaining the stretched muscles for several moments. Your fibers will adjust to the new limits. With an improved flexibility, the risk of experiencing injury will decrease while you are exercising and increasing your performance. Yoga and swimming are some of the exercises that require greater flexibility.

- *Body Composition* - This will show you the percentage of bone, muscles, and fats in your body. These percentages will give you a view on your fitness and health in relation your body's health, age, and weight. Fat and weight are used together most of the time, but the truth is, they're not interchangeable. If you are overweight, it doesn't imply obesity. In fact, there are lots of physically fit people who are overweight because of gaining muscles. But, if you are over fat, you pose health risks that may range to high blood pressure, diabetes, and heart disease.

CHAPTER 2

THE CONDITION OF PEOPLES HEALTH
THESE DAYS

Synopsis

Based from the statements of experts, fitness reflects on one's muscular strength, body composition, and cardio-respiratory endurance.

Some contributors of one's physical wellbeing may include bodyweight management, avoiding unhealthy foods, and proper nutrition. Unfortunately, there is an alarming rate of increasing health risks, which also cause the overall fitness of a person to fail.

There are various factors that reduce the fitness of a person. These factors are as follows:

These Days

Influence

Fitness is said to be influenced by your own actions. Every person has the power to change the level of his or her overall fitness condition through the implementation of changes and by living a healthy and happy lifestyle. Many people will differ when it comes to their fitness level as it depends on the genetics and commitment of each person. Physical activities can help you in various ways and one of these ways is that this can help you avoid certain diseases, obesity, and other health conditions.

Change Your Routine

When working out, it is always essential to make some changes in your routine. One's body needs to keep guessing. This is because if your body is used to your daily routine, this will just result to some issues that may affect your fitness. Take note, altering your daily routine can be the key to your success. For example, if you are doing weight lifting repetitively, it will become much easier for your body to do it. However, if you will add a little twist on your daily exercises, you will surely empower your fitness.

If you are doing exercises for enhancing your cardio, don't just stick on one kind of cardio exercises. Alternate them every week and try other exercises that can contribute on your cardio workout. With this strategy, you won't just be able to increase your fitness, but also your cardio will also boost.

Nutrition

Some people don't realize that eating healthy foods can make a huge difference in increasing the level of your fitness. Whether you aspire to be a runner or you just want to lose weight, picking the right and healthy foods will assist you when making changes on your health. If you are aiming to lose weight, the best way to achieve your goals is by controlling your eating habits. Adding vegetables, grains, and more fruits is best for you. Considering smaller meals will also provide you results in the long run.

If you are having training for racing, the right way to fuel up your body is imperative. You have to get the best amount of carbohydrates and protein for maximum results. Fueling up your body with these minerals will give you more stamina for your race day.

Water

According to a particular health organization, one's body weight is made of sixty percent water. Since the body of a person depends on water, you need to drink enough amount of water to maintain the level of your body fluid even if you have done various activities. Drinking enough amount of water can also help you avoid dehydration, which may cause you to feel tired as you don't have much energy to consume. Water can help you eliminate toxins in your body and transports nutrients to each of your body cells.

Stress

Stress has a lot of effects in one's body. It may cause pains and aches that come from the tense muscles. Stress can also affect your skin. Men may suffer from various sexual problems while women may experience painful menstrual cycle. Heart disease and high blood pressure may also stem from stress. If you are experiencing too much stress, you might not achieve all your goals in fitness.

Alcohol and Drugs

The use of different recreational drugs can cause damage to one's brain cells. You have to take note that the body of each person loses its resistance to several diseases and may cause coordination issues. Alcohol, on the other hand, can cause damage to one's heart, liver, and pancreas. This can also cause increase in health risks and high blood pressure. Both can also affect the mood, memory, and body coordination.

CHAPTER 3

WHAT IS TRUE FITNESS

Synopsis

Fitness means different things. It may mean being able to do various physical activities or it may mean having the right amount of strength and energy. It may also be related to health. Once you get fit, your health will improve.

You don't need to become an athlete for you to get fit. Athletes are required to reach a high level of fitness, and ordinary people only need to walk for a few hours or do several exercises to reach the right fitness level.

Even if you have a busy schedule, you can have the chance to be physically fit. The only thing that you need to know is what fitness is all about and how you can become one of the physically fit individuals.

What Is It

Fitness was defined as the set of attributes, which people achieve or have to do the different physical activities. But, you have to take note that whatever physical activity you're involved with, this does not define the level of your fitness. There are various components of fitness that you must be aware. These components will help you measure your fitness level.

Assessing your fitness level is important, these following components of fitness can be a huge help:

Cardio-Respiratory Endurance

Cardio-respiratory endurance is one's power of his or her respiratory and circulatory systems to generate sufficient energy that will fuel you up in order for you to do all your physical activities. In order for you to boost cardio-respiratory endurance, you need to keep your heart into the safe level that will sustain you when you are walking, running, swimming, bicycling, etc. The activity you prefer doesn't need to be difficult when you are improving cardio-respiratory endurance. If possible, start slowly, and gradually perform on the much intense phase.

Muscular Strength

Muscular strength is one's ability of his or her muscles to exert force during physical activities. The key to make your muscles much stronger is by doing some activities that will let you boost your resistance. If you want to gain muscles and increase your muscle strength, try exercising lifting weights or take stairs rapidly.

Muscular Endurance

This is the ability of the body muscles to continue performing without fatigue. To enhance your muscle endurance, try dancing, walking, bicycling or jogging.

Body Composition

Body composition refers to fat, bone, muscle, and some parts of the body. The total body weight of a person may not change easily time. But, bathroom scales don't assess how much of your body weight contain fats and lean mass. That is the reason why it is essential for you to consider managing your weight.

Flexibility

Flexibility is said to be the motion's range around joints. If you are flexible, you can help you avoid injuries. If you want to boost up flexibility, you must try activities that will test your muscles. Basic stretching programs and swimming can be the best options that you can consider.

CHAPTER 4

WHAT IS THE EMPOWERED
FITNESS MINDSET

Synopsis

For the past few years, the industry of fitness has changed rapidly. High-tech gyms were established and almost everything was changed. However, even if there are lots of things in fitness industry that have gone drastic changes, you must bear in mind that the key to meet all your fitness goals still remain in your mind. Because of this, you need empowered fitness mindset. But, what is empowered fitness mindset all about?

Empowered fitness mindset revolves around having the right mindset to achieve what you want to increase the level of your fitness. At present, it is easy to say that you can do all your goals. But, once you have started to take action, it is never difficult for you to quit than to stay on track. Some people want to be healthy and fit. But, the problem is, they want to do it overnight, which is impossible to achieve as it requires time and effort. There is no quick solution to empower fitness. You must start first by having the right mindset.

There are several factors that affect one's mindset and these are some of them:

The Mindset

- **Motivation** - If you lack strong motivation, the tendency is that you might not be able to reach the things that you want to achieve. If the level of your motivation was high at the very first stage, you must maintain it once you have started your hard work. The reason behind it is that when your motivation level reduced, this will just fail you and you won't get what you want for empowering your fitness. So, seek for the best way to reaffirm your motivation.

- **Remove Fear** - Having fear of not being able to achieve may reduce your confidence. Accepting negativity in yourself may not be a great help as this may just lead you to the wrong path, which is failure. Therefore, if you want to get all your fitness goals, you must stop comparing yourself to other people because you can do better than them.

- **It is More Than a Cardio** - When working out to improve your fitness, overcoming some problems that you will encounter is never been easy. But, this does not mean that you have to give up. Rather than quitting, find ways that will work for you. Try to create some improvements by adapting changes on your lifestyle. Track things including water consumption, nutrition, time spent, body measurements, and sleep times. These things may not be important to you, but they have a huge role in improving the level of your fitness. This will also give you the best mindset in reaching your fitness goals. With this, your confidence will also increase.

- **Seek for a Training Partner or Group** - There are some people who want to have someone that they can count on whenever they are working out. It is because this motivates them. If you are one of those types of persons, then it is wise to seek for a training partner or a group of fitness enthusiasts. This will help you avoid negativity and you will always enjoy working out as the atmosphere is good.

- **Track and Monitor Progress** - Tracking and monitoring progress in all fields of fitness and health will always let you stay on the top of the game. It will also boost your confidence and determination. So, keeping a journal of your daily progress can be helpful.

Giving up is easy especially if you haven't seen any results of your hard work. If you are facing some obstacles when improving your fitness, you must seek for the best way to face such obstacles bravely as this is what empowered fitness mindset all about.

CHAPTER 5

TRADITIONAL FITNESS IDEAS VS. NEW AGE IDEAS

Synopsis

With the advancement of today's technology, there is no wonder that it has also changed the fitness industry. Its impact has brought good and bad things to fitness and the way people aim to increase their level of fitness. However, even if there are new fitness ideas available at present, some still think that traditional fitness ideas are much better. So, what is better between traditional fitness ideas and new age ideas?

What's New

Both traditional fitness ideas and new age ideas have pros and cons. Depending on the preference of a person, he or she can choose between the available ideas in today's market.

Whatever you choose between traditional fitness ideas and new age ideas, the results will still depend on how you worked hard in empowering your fitness.

Traditional fitness ideas rely on using the available gym equipment and having proper nutrition. New age ideas, on the contrary, revolve on using the new concepts of numerous fitness experts by incorporating various approaches, programs, methods, and so on. Both can offer you benefits and may help you increase your fitness level.

New age has brought drastic changes to the fitness industry. Currently, in order for people to get fit, there are available supplements that can be used during workout or while you are under a particular program.

These supplements can be organic and artificial. These types of supplements are proven and effective. However, if you want to be successful with what you want to achieve, you must consider the one that will not fail you and will bring positive effects on your body.

Organic supplements are said to be the best one that you can consider especially if you want to empower your fitness holistically.

When compared to the traditional fitness ideas, new age ideas have opened doors of a wide collection of options. With the available concepts on how to improve one's fitness, you can incorporate a combination of the available ideas in the market today.

You can always any ideas when empowering your fitness. As long as it will keep you on the right track and will give you results in the long run, there is no need to worry about what you have chosen.

Even if there are new ideas for fitness nowadays, traditional fitness ideas still play a huge role in empowering one's fitness as they serve as the foundation of the new age fitness ideas. Without the traditional fitness ideas, new age fitness ideas will not exist.

CHAPTER 6

WHAT DOES EMPOWERMENT FOR FITNESS MEAN TO YOU (HOW TO SET GOALS)

Synopsis

People are always told to think big. Go for gold and reach for the stars. But, when it comes to fitness, you must learn a much calculated approach in order for you to attain your goals effectively. Empowerment for fitness means setting goals that are attainable and much realistic. So, how can you set your fitness goals?

The road to success in empowered fitness is not impossible to reach. The only way you can achieve success is by starting to set your goals. If you don't know how to set goals, here are some of the best ways to do it:

True Fitness For You

- **Take Your Time** - When setting goals for empowering your fitness, you don't need to rush. You can always take your time because you rule on your rules. You just need to focus for you to determine the goals that you want for your fitness.

- **Make Your Goals Specific-** Some people think that resolutions and goals are interchangeable. But, the truth is, resolutions imply that you're deciding something while goals are specific actions, which you want to take. For instance, the phrases "get healthy" is not specific. There are several ways for you to get healthy. This may include stopping smoking, eating the right foods, getting exercises, and so on. If you want a specific goal, you have to define exactly what you really want to do to empower your fitness.

- **Make Your Goals Measurable-** When you are setting goals, you must know how to keep track of your progress. Making this concrete won't only help you to stay on track, but also, this can give you motivation while reaching every step on your milestones.

- **Make Sure That Your Goals are Attainable-** This does not mean that you need to set your bars high just to shoot for the stars. However, there are cases that people set goals that are difficult to attain, which will just lead them to discouragement and failure. This is the reason why there are many people who are giving up when reaching their goals. So, when setting goals, see to it that they are attainable in order for you to avoid anything that will just trigger you to give up.

- **Make Your Goals Much Realistic -** If you are not a runner, running a marathon is an example of unrealistic goal. This does not mean that you can't do one. But, if you want to see to it that your goals are something that you will achieve, you need to asses yourself today to make it more realistic.

- **Set a Time Frame -** Setting a time frame can also be helpful. Without setting a deadline, you won't be motivated in doing your physical activity.

Setting goals wisely can make a difference. But, this may not mean that you will not experience failure. You still need to strive in order for you to achieve success.

CHAPTER 7

WHY ADOPT THE EMPOWERMENT MINDSET FOR FITNESS

Synopsis

The beginnings are always tough, but if you have the right empowerment mindset for fitness, there is no way that you won't achieve all your fitness goals in your set time frame.

That is the reason why you need to consider creating a mindset that will serve as your motivation for achieving your goals. So, why do you need to adopt the right mindset for fitness?

There are many reasons why a proper mindset is important in empowering your fitness. Many people choose to give up when improving their fitness level because they think it is the best way to get rid of the obstacles they are facing. Well, it is true at some point.

But, what they don't know is that giving up will reduce their confidence to try again and reach for the stars.

Being Empowered

It is easy to start achieving your fitness goals, but it is hard to stay on the road most particularly if there are challenging obstacles that you need to face once you have started to do some workout. However, with an empowered mindset for fitness, you can do beyond limits. The reason behind it is that you will be motivated no matter how hard the challenge is.

Another reason why you must adopt empowerment mindset for fitness is that there are cases that some seek for quick fixes for increasing their fitness level. It is not an issue to seek for an easy approach. But, in order for you to achieve success, you must learn in a hard way for you to understand the real meaning of empowerment for fitness.

There are various things that you can consider when adopting empowerment mindset for fitness. First, you need to make sure that you have set goals with the use of your own approach. You may also take for consideration on the different approaches that you can use for setting proper fitness mindset.

However, when creating your own mindset, you need to take note of your needs or preferences. Take note, each person has his or her own wants or needs especially when it comes to leveling up their fitness. If you don't want to fail, you must start by making the right mindset.

Second, you must take actions on your goals. You will never achieve success if you will not start taking actions on your goals. This will serve as the key to the road of success. So, learn the best time to take actions as they may matter in the long run.

There are some reasons why you must adopt empowerment on your mindset for fitness. With this, you will not get healthy. But also, you will have the power to have a defense for diseases or illnesses that may reduce your fitness. So, why wait for a perfect time? Know and understand the reasons behind adopting empowerment mindset for fitness.

CHAPTER 8

TIPS FOR BECOMING EMPOWERED
FOR FITNESS

Synopsis

One of the most essential things that you can do for your fitness is by engaging in various physical activities. Exercising regularly can lower health risks and may improve your overall health and fitness condition. That is the reason why empowering fitness is vital not just for athletes, but also for those who want to avoid illnesses.

There are many ways to become empowered for fitness. If you want to be fit, you can consider the following:

Doing It Right

Aerobic Exercise

Exercises including swimming, walking, bicycling, and jogging can help you strengthen your heart as this will keep you pumping for a long period of time. Aerobic exercise can also assist you in managing your blood pressure and energy levels.

Strength Training

Resistance or strength training can help you build stamina, which will allow you to replace body fats with lean muscle mass that encourage one's body to burn more calories efficiently. This training can also help you counteract those muscles you have lost while doing exercises like pull-ups and pushups.

Fruits and Veggies

A healthy balanced diet, which includes lots of vegetables and fruits can help you promote high levels of physical fitness because they provide the most essential nutrients and minerals to one's body. However, you have to take note that not all vegetables and fruits are healthy and nutritious. That is why you need to pick wisely to get results.

Stretching

In a fitness program, one of the most vital elements is stretching. Stretching can help your body improve your circulation. Stretching can also relieve stress and provides better posture.

Outlook

Healthy diet and regular exercise can help you to empower your fitness. If you consider your personal goals, you will surely get results in the long run. But, before you start your fitness program, you must first consult an expert to know your overall health condition.

CHAPTER 9

THE GOOD AND BAD ABOUT
THE EMPOWERMENT MINDSET FOR FITNESS

Synopsis

Although being physically fit is having a good overall health condition, there are also some advantages and disadvantages that you need to know about empowering fitness. But, even if fitness has its own drawbacks, its benefits still outweigh the bad things about it. For that reason, empowerment mindset for fitness is important.

The Good And Bad

Good Things about Empowerment Mindset for Fitness

The benefits of fitness are many especially if you have incorporated empowerment mindset to reach your goals. These include greater strength, improved appearance, increased energy, better health, more positive mood and attitude, and better health. Some of the benefits of fitness include the following:

1. *Reduces Health Risks* - People who are physically fit can fight against the attack of various diseases or illnesses including the chronic diseases.

2. *Provide Better Health* - Having a high level of fitness can increase both the strength and size of your heart. This will allow your heart to pump more blood, which become more efficient. This will also lower blood pressure and lower pulse, which may increase your lifespan.

3. *Lower the Level of Your Cholesterol* - One of the benefits of empowered fitness is that this can help you control the level of your cholesterol. It can help you reduce the amount of bad cholesterol in your body and maximize the number of good cholesterol.

4. *Build Stronger Ligaments, Joints, and Bones* - If you are physically fit, your muscles will be strengthened. It can also lower the risk of bone diseases. There are also

studies that show that being physically fit can help you reduce osteoporosis' severity.

5. *Improve the Quality of Your Sleep* - One of the main benefits of fitness is that it can help you sleep better. Studies show that those who are regularly exercising can fell asleep easily and they sleep longer compared to those who don't get enough exercise.

There are other benefits of fitness that you will get once you start to take the road of empowered fitness. Overall, fitness can improve the quality of your life and will let you live in a much healthier life.

Bad Things about Empowerment Mindset for Fitness

Although there are many reasons why people consider leveling up their fitness, there are also some problems that may popped up when you start to empower fitness. However, this may depend on the overall health condition of a person.

One of the bad things about empowerment mindset for fitness is that others might not consider following their set deadline when reaching their goals. But, if you have motivation, you can easily avoid it. Another bad thing about it is that some people might choose to give up instead of pursuing their goals. Nevertheless, even if empowerment mindset for fitness may bring negative things for people, its offered benefits are still unbeatable.

CHAPTER 10

CONCLUSION

It is never too late to empower your fitness. As long as you know how to set your fitness goals and you have considered empowerment mindset, you will always keep on the right track. If you want to be successful on your fitness goals, don't forget the things that were mentioned in every chapter. With those things in mind, you won't fail to achieve success.

Empowering fitness does not need to be costly. You won't need money when starting to empower your fitness. All you need is your dedication, determination, focus, and commitment. If you have these qualities, you won't need to worry about failures or mistakes as you will be able to learn how to avoid them. However, even though you have considered everything for empowering your fitness, it does not necessarily mean that you will get empowered fitness without committing mistakes or encountering failures. Depending on what you aim, you must exert efforts as this needs a hundred percent involvement of yourself.

So, what are you waiting for? Don't let yourself suffer from various illnesses or other health risks because you always make a change by taking the road of the new you! Take this challenge now! It is now or never. Take action on your goals and discover the hidden benefits of empowered fitness!

www.ingramcontent.com/pod-product-compliance
Lightning Source LLC
LaVergne TN
LVHW021107090525
810839LV00008B/598